The Nordic Diet

A Beginner's Step-by-Step Guide with Recipes

mf

Disclaimer

By reading this disclaimer, you are accepting the terms of the disclaimer in full. If you disagree with this disclaimer, please do not read the guide.

All of the content within this guide is provided for informational and educational purposes only, and should not be accepted as independent medical or other professional advice. The author is not a doctor, physician, nurse, mental health provider, or registered nutritionist/dietician. Therefore, using and reading this guide does not establish any form of a physician-patient relationship.

Always consult with a physician or another qualified health provider with any issues or questions you might have regarding any sort of medical condition. Do not ever dis- regard any qualified professional medical advice or delay seeking that advice because of anything you have read in this guide. The information in this guide is not intended to be any sort of medical advice and should not be used in lieu of any medical advice by a licensed and qualified medical pro- fessional.

The information in this guide has been compiled from a variety of known sources. However, the author cannot attest to or guarantee the accuracy of each source and thus should not be held liable for any errors or omissions.

Table of Contents

Introduction

The Nordic Diet offers a fresh perspective on food and lifestyle, rooted in the culinary traditions of Northern Europe. This approach celebrates fresh, local, and seasonal ingredients while emphasizing balance, sustainability, and a connection to the land. It's not about strict rules or fad trends—it's about making thoughtful, simple choices that bring both nourishment and joy to the table.

What makes the Nordic Diet truly special is its focus on local produce and ingredients that thrive in their natural seasons. Think of vibrant root vegetables, dark leafy greens, and berries at their peak of flavor. Add to that hearty whole grains like rye and barley, paired with freshly caught seafood, and you have a plate that's as diverse as it is satisfying. By choosing locally grown food, this diet not only delivers exceptional taste but also supports nearby farmers and fosters a sustainable relationship with the environment.

Beyond the delicious ingredients, the Nordic Diet encourages a slower, more mindful way of eating. It's about savoring meals prepared with care, creating connections not just to those who grow the food but also to the people you share it with. This philosophy of sustainability extends to how meals are crafted—reducing waste, respecting natural resources, and making every bite count.

In this guide, we will talk about the following;

- What Is the Nordic Diet?
- Benefits of the Nordic Diet
- 5 Step-by-Step Guide to the Nordic Diet
- Foods to Eat and Foods to Limit
- What Sets the Nordic Diet Apart?
- 7-Day Sample Meal Plan
- Sample Recipes

Keep reading to learn more about the Nordic Diet and discover how it can transform your relationship with food for the better. By the end of this guide, you'll have all the tools and knowledge you need to embark on your own Nordic Diet journey and start reaping its many benefits.

What Is the Nordic Diet?

The Nordic Diet is more than just a way of eating—it's a lifestyle inspired by the traditions and values of the Nordic region, which includes Sweden, Norway, Denmark, Iceland, and Finland. These countries stand out for their progressive approach to well-being, and their people are often heralded as some of the happiest in the world. This connection between culture and happiness has drawn global attention, inspiring many to adopt Nordic principles in their own lives.

Central to this influence are the philosophies of hygge, lagom, and friluftsliv, which reflect the Nordic ethos of balance, sustainability, and a strong connection to nature. These concepts shape the backbone of the Nordic Diet:

- *Hygge*, a hallmark of Danish culture, embodies a sense of coziness, warmth, and contentment. Picture enjoying a hearty meal with loved ones in a calm, inviting atmosphere.
- *Lagom*, a Swedish term meaning "just the right amount," emphasizes moderation. It's about balancing

indulgence and restraint, finding satisfaction without overdoing or depriving yourself.

- *Friluftsliv* translates to "open-air life" in Norwegian and Swedish. It encourages a deep appreciation for nature and outdoor living, showing how restorative activities like hiking or picnicking enhance health and happiness.

These principles seamlessly merge into the Nordic Diet, offering a holistic approach that goes beyond food.

At its heart, the Nordic Diet champions simplicity, sustainability, and a return to natural ingredients. Its core practices include:

- *Eating more plant-based foods:* Such as root vegetables, berries, nuts, legumes, and whole grains, provides essential vitamins, minerals, and fiber while reducing reliance on meat. Shifting to a plant-based diet can also support heart health and help lower your environmental impact.
- *Including foods from lakes and oceans:* Like fish, shellfish, and seaweed, ensures your body gets essential nutrients like omega-3 fatty acids, iodine, and high-quality protein. These foods are not only nutritious but also key to maintaining brain and heart health.
- *Choosing local, seasonal, and organic produce:* Helps you get the freshest, most nutrient-dense food available while supporting local farmers. Seasonal eating also

reduces the carbon footprint of your diet and aligns with the natural growing cycles of your region.

- *Using canola oil:* A versatile and heart-healthy option, is rich in omega-3 fatty acids and low in saturated fats, making it a great choice for both cooking and salad dressings. It's an easy way to incorporate healthier fats into your meals.

- *Avoiding processed foods:* Refined grains, and artificial additives allows you to focus on natural, wholesome options that nourish your body. Processed foods often contain added sugars, unhealthy fats, and preservatives, which can negatively impact your health over time.

- *Minimizing waste:* By adopting a mindful, eco-conscious approach to cooking and shopping involves buying only what you need, repurposing leftovers, and composting food scraps whenever possible. This not only reduces your environmental footprint but also saves money and inspires creativity in the kitchen.

The Nordic Diet isn't about strict rules or fad-driven restrictions. It's a flexible framework that connects your plate to nature, your community, and your well-being. It invites you to enjoy nourishing meals that align with the rhythm of the seasons while fostering an enduring respect for the environment.

Benefits of the Nordic Diet

The Nordic Diet is more than an eating plan—it's a lifestyle that prioritizes natural, nutrient-rich foods, with benefits that extend far beyond the plate. Centered on fruits, vegetables, whole grains, nuts, seeds, fish, and seafood, this diet delivers a powerful combination of nutrients and fiber essential for overall well-being.

Nutrient-Rich Eating Made Simple

By focusing on locally sourced and seasonal ingredients, the Nordic Diet provides a wealth of antioxidants, vitamins, minerals, and fiber. These nutrients play a key role in supporting immunity, improving digestion, and maintaining energy.

Instead of opting for processed foods filled with added sugars and unhealthy fats, the diet promotes fresh, wholesome options like berries, root vegetables, pulses, and whole grains. This shift not only makes eating healthier but also tastier and more enjoyable.

A Natural Approach to Weight Management

One of the standout benefits of the Nordic Diet is its ability to aid in weight management. The focus on high-fiber foods and lean proteins helps keep you full longer, reducing the temptation to overeat.

Evidence backs up its effectiveness. A study involving 147 overweight participants found that those following the Nordic Diet lost an average of 4.7 kg compared to only 1.5 kg in those on a typical Danish diet. Another six-week study showed participants shed 5% of their total body weight without any calorie restrictions or additional exercise.

Beyond weight loss, the diet targets abdominal fat, a key risk factor for metabolic conditions like type-2 diabetes. By maintaining a healthier weight and forming better eating habits, practitioners lower their risk of chronic diseases while enjoying long-term results.

Lower Risk of Chronic Diseases

The Nordic Diet helps improve heart health, regulate blood pressure, and stabilize blood sugar levels. A seven-month study demonstrated that obese participants experienced reductions in both systolic (5.1 mmHg) and diastolic (3.2 mmHg) blood pressure when following this eating style. Additionally, it curbs LDL or "bad" cholesterol, which contributes to heart disease and stroke risks. These preventative benefits extend to conditions like diabetes and even cancer.

Fighting Chronic Inflammation

Chronic inflammation in the body is a known precursor to conditions such as hypertension, diabetes, and cancer. The Nordic Diet naturally combats inflammation by emphasizing anti-inflammatory foods like fish, whole grains, fresh vegetables, fruits, and heart-healthy fats from canola oil. Paired with regular physical activity and adequate sleep, this anti-inflammatory approach not only extends life expectancy but enhances quality of life.

Promoting Sustainability and Mindful Choices

The Nordic Diet goes beyond personal health by advocating for environmental well-being. It encourages the use of seasonal, organic, and locally sourced produce, which minimizes carbon footprints and supports community agriculture. The approach stresses reducing meat consumption and making mindful food choices, such as favoring responsibly sourced fish and meat.

Home-cooked meals are another core element, shifting focus away from convenience foods. This encourages mindful eating—enjoying meals slowly, savoring every bite, and fostering a deeper connection to food. By minimizing food waste and prioritizing sustainable practices, the Nordic Diet aligns with both individual and environmental wellness.

Taking on the Nordic Diet doesn't mean rigid rules or deprivation. Instead, it's about forming habits that prioritize health, flavor, and sustainability. Adopting this lifestyle can make a meaningful difference not only to your health but to the planet as well.

5 Step-by-Step Guide to the Nordic Diet

The Nordic Diet is a refreshing and wholesome way to eat that embraces local, seasonal ingredients and simple cooking methods. Here's how you can make it a part of your lifestyle, one step at a time.

Step 1: Shift to Whole, Seasonal Foods

The first and most important step in adopting the Nordic Diet is making seasonal, whole foods the star of your kitchen. Not only are these foods loaded with flavor and nutrients, but they also align beautifully with sustainable living. By focusing on what's in season, you're not only nourishing your body but also supporting local farmers and reducing the environmental impact of your meals.

Why Eat Seasonally?

Seasonal produce is at its peak flavor, freshness, and nutritional value. For example, strawberries in summer are sweeter and juicier compared to those grown out of season, and winter vegetables like cabbage or kale are heartier when grown in the colder months. Eating what's in season also reduces the carbon footprint of your meals since you're avoiding food that's been transported across the globe. Plus, seasonal items are usually more affordable because they're in abundance.

Shopping for Seasonal Foods

Start by visiting your local farmer's market to explore fresh, local produce. This is one of the best ways to connect with what's growing in your area. Farmers are often happy to share cooking tips or suggest how to use lesser-known vegetables like celeriac or rutabaga. If you can't visit a farmer's market, consider joining a CSA (Community Supported Agriculture) program. These subscriptions provide you with a weekly box of locally harvested produce—and often include seasonal surprises that encourage you to try new recipes.

At the grocery store, read labels carefully. Look for terms like "locally grown" or produce that lists a nearby farm as the source. Imported, out-of-season items might be tempting, but sticking to local options makes all the difference in building an environmentally friendly and nutrient-rich diet.

Meal Planning Around Seasonal Ingredients

When you build your meals, think about which vegetables, fruits, and herbs are at their best during the current season. For example:

1. *Spring*

Spring brings a bounty of fresh, vibrant flavors. Incorporate asparagus, spinach, and radishes into your cooking to celebrate the season. For a quick and refreshing meal, try making a light spring salad with tender spinach leaves, crisp radish slices, and a simple olive oil dressing. You can also roast asparagus with a sprinkle of sea salt for a healthy side dish or use it in a creamy risotto.

2. *Summer*

Summer is the perfect time to enjoy zucchini, tomatoes, and berries at their peak. Take advantage of the abundance of zucchini by grilling slices with a touch of olive oil and herbs or spiralizing it into a zucchini noodle dish. Juicy tomatoes are perfect for caprese salads or homemade tomato sauce. For a sweet treat, top your whole-grain oatmeal with fresh strawberries, blueberries, or raspberries for a breakfast that feels like dessert.

3. *Fall*

Fall is all about earthy, comforting flavors like pumpkins, parsnips, sweet potatoes, and hearty greens. Roasted root vegetable bowls are a delicious and versatile option—combine pumpkin, parsnips, and sweet potatoes with quinoa, and finish with a drizzle of canola oil or a tahini-based dressing. Don't forget to use hearty greens like kale or Swiss chard in soups, casseroles, or sautéed as a side dish. And of course, pumpkin puree is perfect for baking everything from muffins to pies!

4. *Winter*

Winter's chill calls for comforting, hearty meals featuring root vegetables like carrots, turnips, and cabbage. Warm up with dishes like a cabbage and apple slaw spiced with cinnamon and apple cider vinegar, perfect as a side or light meal. Or try a creamy carrot-parsnip soup that's both nourishing and satisfying. You can also roast turnips with garlic and rosemary for a simple yet flavorful addition to your winter menu.

Reducing Processed Foods

A key part of this step is moving away from processed and pre-packaged items. These often contain additives, excess sodium, and unhealthy fats that can derail your health and the simplicity of the Nordic Diet. Instead, opt for natural, unprocessed ingredients that you can see and identify—like whole potatoes instead of instant mash.

Transitioning away from processed foods can feel overwhelming at first, so make small swaps. For example, replace sugary breakfast cereals with steel-cut oats topped with seasonal fruit. Swap frozen, breaded fish fillets for fresh salmon or cod. The trick is to gradually rebuild your meals so they're made up of whole, fresh ingredients.

Practical Tips to Start Shifting

- *Batch Cooking:* Prep several seasonal ingredients ahead of time. Roast a variety of root veggies on Sunday to use as sides or in salads throughout the week.
- *Herb Garden:* Start with basic herbs like parsley, dill, and chives that are commonly used in Nordic recipes. They're easy to grow on a balcony or windowsill and add freshness to your meals.
- *Keep It Simple:* Seasonal eating doesn't mean you need fancy recipes. A humble plate of potatoes, baked salmon, and steamed kale with a squeeze of lemon is a nutritious and satisfying meal.

By prioritizing whole, seasonal foods, you're reconnecting with natural eating habits that are central to the Nordic Diet. Beyond improving your health, this approach invites you to celebrate what nature has to offer, one season at a time.

Step 2: Focus on Healthy Fats

Healthy fats are an essential component of the Nordic Diet, and they play a vital role in keeping your heart, brain, and overall body in top form. These fats come from natural sources like fatty fish, plant-based oils, nuts, and seeds. Unlike unhealthy fats found in processed foods or deep-fried meals, healthy fats deliver a dose of nutrients without compromising your well-being. Here's how to include them in your diet effectively.

The Benefits of Healthy Fats

Including healthy fats in your meals contributes to better health in several ways. Omega-3 fatty acids, found in fatty fish like salmon and mackerel, are known for reducing inflammation, supporting brain function, and lowering the risk of heart disease. Plant-based fats, such as those found in canola oil, walnuts, and flaxseeds, also support cardiovascular health while providing essential nutrients like vitamin E and healthy lipids for sustained energy.

Choosing Healthy Fats

To harness these benefits, prioritize fats from natural, nutrient-dense sources:

- *Fatty Fish:* Salmon, mackerel, herring, trout, and sardines are excellent choices. These fish are rich in omega-3s and provide high-quality protein.
- *Plant-Based Oils:* Canola oil is a Nordic favorite because of its mild flavor and versatility. Olive oil is another great option for salads and low-heat cooking.
- *Nuts and Seeds:* Add a handful of walnuts, almonds, flaxseeds, or chia seeds to your meals. These provide a satisfying crunch along with healthy fats.

At the same time, reduce your intake of less nutritious fats by replacing butter, margarine, and highly processed oils with these healthier options.

Incorporating More Healthy Fats Into Meals

There are simple yet delicious ways to boost your intake of healthy fats throughout the day:

- *Breakfast:* Add a drizzle of canola oil to whole-grain oatmeal and top it with flaxseeds or omega-rich walnuts. Alternatively, spread ripe avocado on whole-grain rye bread.
- *Lunch:* Create a Nordic-inspired salad with leafy greens, smoked salmon, a sprinkle of sunflower seeds, and a light dressing made from canola or olive oil, lemon juice, and dill.
- *Dinner:* Bake salmon or mackerel with a lemon-dill marinade, and pair it with roasted Brussels sprouts tossed in canola oil. Or, make a hearty trout stew with root vegetables.
- *Snacks:* Opt for a small handful of almonds or a rye crispbread topped with avocado and a sprinkle of chia seeds.

Cooking Tips to Preserve Nutritional Value

When working with healthy fats, it's important to use cooking methods that maintain their nutritional properties. High heat can degrade some plant-based oils, like olive oil, reducing their benefits. Here's how to keep your dishes both healthy and flavorful:

- *Low and Slow:* Use low to medium heat when sautéing or cooking with plant-based oils to preserve their quality.
- *Baking and Roasting:* Coating fish or vegetables in canola oil before baking or roasting helps bring out flavors while keeping nutrients intact.
- *Steaming:* Pair steamed vegetables with a drizzle of olive oil or a dollop of nut butter for a nutritious boost.
- *Dressings and Sauces:* Use oils cold in salad dressings, dips, or marinades to retain their nutritional value.

Reducing Unhealthy Fats

Making the switch from less healthy fats to healthier versions can take time. A good approach is to find direct swaps that work for your palate and lifestyle:

- Replace butter on your toast with a spread of mashed avocado or nut butter.
- Swap deep-fried fish for baked herring or salmon fillets with a crispy whole-grain breadcrumb coating.
- Use canola or olive oil for sautéing rather than margarine or vegetable shortening.

A Nordic-Inspired Menu Idea

For a day filled with healthy fats, try this Nordic-inspired meal plan:

- *Breakfast:* Rye toast with avocado and smoked salmon.
- *Lunch:* A salad of kale, barley, grilled trout, and a canola oil vinaigrette.
- *Snack:* Yogurt with a drizzle of flaxseed oil and fresh blueberries.
- *Dinner:* Oven-baked salmon with roasted root vegetables, dressed with a light olive oil drizzle.

By focusing on healthy fats, you're fueling your body with nutrients it craves. This step of the Nordic Diet isn't just about adding omega-rich foods; it's about shifting your mindset toward balance and wellness. Little by little, with each meal prepared thoughtfully, you'll build a habit that improves both your health and your enjoyment of wholesome, satisfying dishes.

Step 3: Make Whole Grains Your Base

Whole grains are a vital part of the Nordic Diet, offering a hearty, nutritious foundation for your meals. They are unrefined, packed with fiber, and loaded with essential nutrients that support your health and keep you energized throughout the day. By making whole grains like rye, barley, and oats your base, you'll be fueling your body with slow-digesting carbs that provide lasting energy while promoting better digestion.

The Benefits of Whole Grains

Whole grains are far superior to refined grains (like white bread or regular pasta). They offer:

- *Improved digestion:* Thanks to their high fiber content, whole grains help maintain gut health and regular bowel movements.
- *Sustained energy:* The complex carbohydrates in rye, barley, and oats break down slowly, keeping you fuller for longer and avoiding blood sugar spikes.
- *Heart health:* Whole grains can help lower cholesterol levels and reduce the risk of heart disease.
- *Rich nutrients:* They're packed with vitamins, minerals, and antioxidants like B vitamins, magnesium, iron, and selenium.

Choosing Whole Grains for the Nordic Diet

When planning your meals, opt for hearty, nutrient-dense grains. Here are some staples of the Nordic Diet and ideas on how to use them:

- *Rye:* Look for dense rye bread at your local bakery or try baking your own. It's perfect for open-faced sandwiches topped with smoked salmon, avocado, or a light cheese. You can also snack on rye crispbread for a crunchy, fiber-rich treat.

- *Barley:* Use barley in soups, stews, or grain bowls. Its chewy texture and nutty flavor make it an excellent alternative to rice or quinoa. Barley also works great as a base for a warm grain salad with roasted vegetables and a drizzle of olive oil.
- *Oats:* Start your morning with a bowl of whole-grain oats. You can top them with fresh berries, nuts, and a spoonful of honey for a delicious and nutrient-rich breakfast. Alternatively, bake them into homemade muesli or granola for a versatile snack.
- *Other Options:* Incorporate spelt, buckwheat, or whole-grain rye flour into your baking for a Nordic-inspired flair.

At the same time, aim to reduce your intake of refined grains, such as white bread, pastries, and standard pasta. Gradually transitioning to whole-grain alternatives ensures you won't feel overwhelmed as you adjust to this healthier way of eating.

Incorporating Whole Grains into Your Meals

Adding whole grains to every meal is simple with a few tweaks:

- *Breakfast:* Swap out sugary cereals for oatmeal cooked with water or milk. Stir in warming spices like cinnamon and nutmeg, and garnish with apples, blueberries, or flaxseeds.

- **Lunch:** Prepare an open-faced sandwich on rye bread. Top it with avocado, mashed chickpeas, or smoked herring for a Nordic twist. You can also make a barley and vegetable soup for a warming midday meal.
- **Dinner:** Serve hearty entrees with a whole-grain base. For instance, try barley risotto with mushrooms, or pair baked salmon with a side of steamed spinach and a serving of whole-grain rye berry salad.
- **Snacks:** Keep it simple with rye crackers spread with light cream cheese or hummus. Alternatively, bake whole-grain muffins using spelt or oat flour and add seasonal ingredients like grated carrots or cranberries.

Cooking Methods to Enhance Flavor and Texture

Cooking whole grains properly is key to enjoying their unique textures and flavors:

- **Pre-Soaking:** Barley and other hearty grains benefit from soaking before cooking. This softens the husk and reduces cooking time.
- **Simmering:** Use a ratio of 3 cups liquid to 1 cup of grain for most grains like barley or rye berries. Cooking in vegetable stock instead of water can add extra flavor.
- **Roasting:** For a nutty depth of flavor, toast grains like oats or barley lightly in a dry pan before cooking.

- *Mixing Grains:* Combine different grains like barley, rye berries, and spelt for added texture and flavor in salads and bowls.

Reducing Refined Grains

Transitioning from refined grains to whole grains is easier than you might think. Start by replacing white breads and crackers with rye bread and crispbreads. Instead of white or instant rice, try cooking barley, farro, or bulgur as a side dish. Gradually incorporate more oatmeal or muesli into your breakfasts instead of sugary cereals or pastries.

A Nordic-Inspired Whole-Grain Menu Idea

Here's an idea for a menu featuring whole grains:

- *Breakfast:* Warm oatmeal topped with lingonberry jam, crushed almonds, and a splash of milk.
- *Lunch:* Barley salad with roasted beets, crumbled goat cheese, and a drizzle of dill vinaigrette.
- *Snack:* Rye crispbread with cream cheese and thinly sliced cucumbers.
- *Dinner:* Hearty vegetable stew served with freshly baked rye bread on the side.

Making whole grains the base of your meals not only boosts your health but also celebrates one of the cornerstones of Nordic cuisine. Over time, you'll come to appreciate the robust flavors and satisfying texture that these grains bring to your table. By swapping out refined options, you're making a meaningful step toward a healthier you!

Step 4: Eat More Plant-Based Meals

Plant-based meals are an essential pillar of the Nordic Diet, offering countless benefits for both your health and the environment. While this diet includes moderate amounts of meat and fish, a significant emphasis is placed on vegetables, legumes, and other plant-based ingredients as the foundation of your meals. By shifting the focus to plants, you'll not only unlock a rainbow of flavors and textures but also enjoy a diet that's rich in nutrients.

The Benefits of Plant-Based Eating

- *Better health:* A diet rich in vegetables and legumes is associated with lower risks of heart disease, Type 2 diabetes, and certain cancers. These foods are loaded with vitamins, minerals, fiber, and antioxidants that strengthen your body.
- *Environmentally friendly:* Eating more plant-based foods reduces your carbon footprint, as plant production generally requires fewer resources than livestock farming.
- *Supports weight management:* Plant-based meals are often lower in calories yet high in fiber, keeping you satisfied for longer without overeating.

Plant-Based Ingredients to Focus On

- *Vegetables:* Root vegetables like carrots, parsnips, and beets are staples of Nordic cuisine. Incorporate cruciferous vegetables such as cabbage, broccoli, and Brussels sprouts, along with dark leafy greens like kale and spinach.
- *Legumes:* Beans, lentils, and peas are excellent sources of protein and fiber. Lentils cook quickly, making them perfect for weeknight meals, while dried peas and beans are great for soups and stews.
- *Whole Grains:* Barley, rye, and oats can complement plant-based meals by adding bulk and texture.
- *Nuts and seeds:* Sunflower seeds, flaxseeds, and hazelnuts are common in Nordic diets. Sprinkle them over salads or oatmeal for added crunch and nutrients.
- *Herbs and spices:* Add flavor and depth to your meals with fresh dill, parsley, or thyme. Spices like caraway and mustard seeds are also popular in Nordic-inspired dishes.

Balancing Plant-Based Meals with Animal Proteins

The Nordic Diet doesn't call for cutting out meat entirely but advocates for its thoughtful use. Aim to keep meat as an accent rather than the star. For example:

- Mix lentils or mushrooms into minced meats in recipes like meatballs or casseroles to reduce the portion of meat while boosting plant content.

- Use fish, particularly fatty types like salmon or mackerel, as occasional protein sources to complement plant-based staples.

Ideas for Plant-Based Nordic Meals

Here's how you can build flavorful and satisfying plant-based plates while sticking to Nordic principles:

- *Breakfast:* Enjoy an open-faced sandwich on rye bread topped with smashed avocado, sliced radishes, and a sprinkle of sunflower seeds.
- *Lunch:* Whip up a hearty lentil and vegetable soup with carrots, celery, and Nordic spices like dill or caraway. Add a slice of rye crispbread on the side.
- *Dinner:* Serve roasted root vegetables—like beets, parsnips, and sweet potatoes—as the centerpiece, paired with a creamy dill yogurt sauce. Add a small portion of barley or quinoa to round out the meal.
- *Snacks:* Try hummus or pea spread with rye crackers. Or make a quick salad from shredded carrots, cabbage, and apple, tossed with a mustard vinaigrette.

Tips for Enhancing Flavor and Nutrition

- *Roasting:* Roasting vegetables at high heat brings out natural sweetness and enhances flavor. Drizzle vegetables like carrots, broccoli, or squash with olive oil, season with salt and pepper, then roast until caramelized.

- *Fermentation:* Incorporate fermented veggies, like sauerkraut, for a boost of gut-friendly probiotics and unique tangy flavors.
- *Blending:* Make hearty purees or soups from vegetables such as pumpkin, cauliflower, or peas. Blend cooked veggies with a bit of veggie broth for a creamy consistency.
- *Marination:* Marinate vegetables like zucchini or mushrooms with olive oil, garlic, and fresh herbs before grilling or baking them. This adds rich layers of flavor.
- *Batch cooking:* Prepare beans and lentils in large batches and store portions in the fridge or freezer. This makes it easy to incorporate legumes into meals during busy weeks.

Transitioning to Plant-Based Meals

Start small by making gradual changes:

- Dedicate one or two days a week to meatless meals. Build filling and satisfying plant-based options that you love.
- Swap out common animal proteins for legumes. For example, replace chicken in a stew with chickpeas, or try black beans instead of ground beef in tacos.
- Use vegetables creatively in place of refined or processed ingredients. For instance, make cabbage wraps instead of tortillas or use roasted cauliflower steaks as a centerpiece instead of meat.

A Simple Nordic-Inspired Plant-Based Menu

- *Breakfast:* Porridge made from oats, topped with seasonal berries, a drizzle of maple syrup, and a handful of hazelnuts.
- *Lunch:* Kale, cabbage, and lentil salad with a mustard-dill dressing. Add some roasted root vegetables for a bit of sweetness and texture.
- *Snack:* Rye crispbread with pea puree or mashed avocado sprinkled with fresh dill.
- *Dinner:* Hearty roasted vegetables (parsnips, carrots, and Brussels sprouts) with spelt or barley, drizzled with a creamy tahini dressing.

By making vegetables, legumes, and other plant-based ingredients a larger part of your plate, you'll not only nurture your health but also enjoy delicious, wholesome meals. The Nordic Diet's flexibility allows you to strike a balance between plant-based eating and moderate use of animal protein, ensuring your diet is both fulfilling and sustainable.

Step 5: Keep It Simple and Homemade

Cooking from scratch is at the heart of the Nordic Diet's philosophy. By focusing on simple, wholesome techniques like boiling, baking, and roasting, you can create meals that are both nourishing and flavorful. The Nordic approach is all about letting the natural ingredients shine without masking them with heavy sauces or additives. This not only supports your health but also fosters a deeper connection to the food you eat.

The Benefits of Cooking from Scratch

- **Better control over ingredients:** When you prepare meals at home, you choose what goes into them, avoiding hidden sugars, unhealthy fats, or excessive salt often found in processed foods.
- **Improved nutrition:** Homemade meals often have more vitamins, minerals, and fiber since you're using fresh, whole ingredients.
- **Balanced portions:** Cooking for yourself allows you to control serving sizes and ensure your plate is filled with nutrient-dense foods.
- **Healthier habits:** Cooking at home encourages mindful eating and often leads to a more sustainable, balanced diet over time.
- **Connection with food:** Preparing food from scratch strengthens your bond with ingredients and brings mindfulness to cooking and eating.

Simple Cooking Techniques to Elevate Natural Flavors

The beauty of the Nordic Diet lies in its simplicity. Here are classic cooking techniques to enhance the flavor of fresh, seasonal ingredients:

Boiling: A gentle way to cook vegetables, grains, or fish while preserving their nutrients and flavors. For example:

- Boil root vegetables like carrots, potatoes, and parsnips until tender, then toss them with a small amount of olive oil and fresh dill.
- Use boiling to prepare whole grains like barley or rye berries. Add a pinch of salt and cook until chewy and nutty.

Baking: Baking is an easy method that requires minimal effort while delivering rich, concentrated flavors:

- Bake whole-grain breads, such as rye or spelt loaves, which are staples in the Nordic Diet.
- Roast your favorite vegetables, like beets, sweet potatoes, and cauliflower, for a caramelized and naturally sweet taste. Drizzle olive oil over them, sprinkle with herbs, and bake until golden.

Roasting: Roasting meat, fish, or root vegetables at high temperatures intensifies flavors and adds texture.

- Roast a whole fillet of salmon with a touch of sea salt, lemon, and fresh dill for a Nordic-inspired protein centerpiece.
- Spread chickpeas on a baking tray with a little oil, paprika, and salt for a crunchy snack or salad topping.

Stewing: A classic way to create hearty, comforting meals that last for several days:

- Prepare a Nordic-style vegetable soup with barley, carrots, cabbage, and leeks. Season with caraway seeds and garnish with fresh parsley.

Practical Tips for Meal Prepping

Bringing the simplicity of the Nordic Diet into your routine can be easier when you plan ahead. Meal prepping ensures you have healthy options available, even during busy days. Here's how to do it:

- *Batch cook soups and stews:* Prepare several servings of a nutrient-packed soup or stew over the weekend. Store portions in the refrigerator or freeze for later. For example, a barley and vegetable soup with root vegetables and fresh herbs makes a perfect lunch or dinner base.
- *Roast vegetables in bulk:* Make a tray of mixed vegetables (carrots, sweet potatoes, onions) that you can use throughout the week as a side dish, salad topping, or snack.
- *Bake whole-grain breads or crackers:* Spend time baking rye bread or crispbreads that will keep well and provide a healthy carb option throughout the week.
- *Prepare grain bases:* Cook larger portions of barley, quinoa, or rye berries to use in various meals. These can be stored in the fridge and reheated as needed.

Avoiding Processed Foods and Heavy Sauces

An essential aspect of the Nordic Diet is minimizing processed foods and artificial ingredients. Instead, opt for pure, whole ingredients. Tips for bypassing overly processed choices include:

- *Read labels:* Look for short ingredient lists with items you recognize when buying packaged foods like bread or crackers.
- *Make your own sauces and condiments:* Avoid store-bought dressings or heavy creams filled with preservatives. For instance, prepare a simple dressing from mustard, dill, olive oil, and vinegar.
- *Choose natural sweeteners:* If you need sweetness, use small amounts of honey or maple syrup instead of refined sugar.

Enjoying the Cooking Process

Cooking doesn't have to feel like a chore. It can become a meaningful part of your day that brings joy and creativity into your life. Here are ways to make it an enjoyable experience:

- *Create a calming environment:* Play your favorite music, light a candle, or sip on tea while you cook.
- *Get inspired by nature:* Take note of seasonal produce to help guide your meals. A trip to a farmer's market might spark new ideas.

- *Cook with others:* Invite family or friends to cook with you. Sharing a homemade meal is a wonderful way to connect.
- *Celebrate simplicity:* Remember, you don't need fancy recipes or equipment. A few high-quality ingredients can go a long way in creating a satisfying dish.

By following these steps, you'll gradually adopt the Nordic Diet in a practical, sustainable way. It's about celebrating nature's bounty while treating your body well—so enjoy the simplicity and richness this diet brings to your table!

The Nordic Diet is inspired by the traditional eating habits of Nordic countries like Denmark, Finland, Iceland, Norway, and Sweden. It emphasizes whole, locally-sourced, and sustainable foods. Here's a breakdown of what to eat and what to avoid:

Foods to Eat

To follow the Nordic Diet, focus on incorporating these foods into your meals:

1. **Fruits and Vegetables**

   Focus on seasonal and locally-sourced produce. Berries, root vegetables, and cabbage are staples.

2. **Whole Grains**

   Include oats, rye, and barley. These grains are often consumed in bread, porridge, and other dishes.

3. Fish and Seafood

Rich in omega-3 fatty acids, fish like salmon, herring, and mackerel are central to the diet.

4. Legumes

Beans and peas are encouraged for their protein and fiber content.

5. Nuts and Seeds

These are good sources of healthy fats and protein.

6. Dairy

Low-fat options like skyr (a type of yogurt) and cheese are included.

7. Herbs and Spices

Dill, parsley, and mustard are commonly used for flavoring.

8. Healthy Fats

Use canola oil and other plant-based oils instead of butter.

By incorporating these foods into your meals, you'll be nourishing your body with a balanced and diverse array of nutrients. Not only that, but you'll also be supporting local farmers and reducing your carbon footprint by choosing locally-sourced options.

Foods to Limit

While the Nordic Diet is flexible and not strictly restrictive, it's important to limit consumption of these foods:

1. **Red Meat**

   This includes beef, pork, and lamb. They can be consumed in moderation but are not a central part of the diet.

2. **Processed Foods**

   These include pre-packaged snacks, frozen meals, and highly processed meats like bacon and sausages.

3. **Sugary Foods**

   Limit your intake of added sugars from sources like candy, pastries, and sugary beverages.

4. **Salt**

   Aim to reduce salt intake by limiting processed foods and using herbs and spices for flavor instead.

5. **Alcohol**

   While some Nordic countries have a culture of drinking alcohol with meals, it's recommended to limit consumption for health reasons. Opt for red wine in moderation, as it has been shown to have some health benefits.

By limiting these foods, you'll be further promoting a healthy and balanced diet that supports your overall well-being.

What Sets the Nordic Diet Apart?

The Nordic Diet has garnered widespread acclaim for its ability to improve health, promote sustainable eating practices, and inspire lasting lifestyle changes. While many compare it to the Mediterranean Diet due to their shared focus on wholesome, plant-based foods and healthy fats, the Nordic Diet distinguishes itself through its principles and practices. This chapter explores how the Nordic Diet stands out from other dietary frameworks, dispels common myths, and highlights its unique advantages.

How the Nordic Diet Compares to Other Diets

The comparisons between the Nordic Diet and other popular eating plans like the Mediterranean Diet are inevitable, given their shared focus on heart-healthy ingredients and minimally processed foods. However, the Nordic Diet sets itself apart in key ways:

1. **A Strong Focus on Local, Seasonal, and Organic Foods**

   Unlike most diets, the Nordic Diet insists on prioritizing food that is locally grown, responsibly sourced, and in season. While Mediterranean cuisine often highlights olive oil, tomatoes, and citrus fruits that thrive in its sunny climate, Nordic cuisine adapts to a colder, more temperate region.

   This leads to the use of ingredients that are more sustainable for the local environment, such as root vegetables (like turnips or carrots), cabbage, and a wide variety of berries.

   By encouraging the consumption of locally grown produce, the diet isn't just healthier—it's also more eco-friendly and cost-effective. Seasonal produce tends to be fresher, more flavorful, and less expensive than imported foods, making it easier for people to eat healthy on a budget.

2. **The Health Benefits of Canola Oil**

   Perhaps the Nordic Diet's most notable divergence from other diets is its emphasis on canola (rapeseed) oil as the primary cooking fat. While the Mediterranean Diet champions olive oil, canola oil boasts its own compelling health benefits.

   Rich in monounsaturated fats and with the lowest levels of saturated fats among vegetable oils, it is a heart-healthy choice for reducing cholesterol and inflammation. Canola also contains a higher proportion of omega-3 fatty acids compared to olive oil, further supporting cardiovascular and brain health.

Research has consistently shown that canola oil's nutrient profile is particularly suited to improving metabolic markers such as blood pressure and insulin sensitivity. Plus, its neutral flavor makes it versatile, lending itself well to Nordic recipes without overpowering the taste of natural ingredients.

3. Whole Grains and Foraged Foods

While many diets advocate for whole grains, the Nordic Diet takes it to another level by emphasizing grains that are less common outside the Nordic region. Foods like rye and barley, for instance, are often overlooked in other diets yet serve as staples in the Nordic food plan. These grains are particularly high in nutrients like fiber, B vitamins, and magnesium, all of which contribute to better digestion and heart health.

Another fascinating feature of the Nordic Diet is the inclusion of foraged foods. Mushrooms, moss, wild herbs, flower petals, and fresh berries are used to add diversity and nutrition to meals. Foraging encourages a deeper connection to nature and enhances sustainability, as it reduces reliance on commercially farmed foods.

Unique Advantages of the Nordic Diet

The Nordic Diet offers unique benefits that go beyond the obvious. By making certain nutritional and practical choices, it provides advantages in areas where other diets may fall short.

1. *Sustainability and Environmental Friendliness:* By emphasizing local food systems and discouraging food waste, the Nordic Diet is aligned with environmental sustainability. It recognizes the importance of reducing the carbon footprint of imported goods and overfarmed crops, instead encouraging people to cook with what's naturally available in their region.

2. *A Balanced Blend of Traditions and Modern Health Science:* Nordic cuisine draws inspiration from ancient food practices yet is shaped by cutting-edge nutritional research. This blend ensures that meals derived from this plan are both deeply rooted in tradition and highly effective at reducing modern risks like heart disease, obesity, diabetes, and chronic inflammation.

3. *Adaptability for Weight Management:* Many people struggle with diets that feel overly restrictive. The Nordic Diet makes healthy eating easier and more sustainable by allowing for indulgence in flavorful recipes like fish stews, berry desserts, and hearty rye breads. Studies indicate that calorie density tends to be lower in Nordic-inspired meals, making it easier for

people to naturally achieve weight control without constant calorie-counting.

4. *A Holistic Approach to Food and Wellness:* Nordic eating isn't just about the nutrients—it's a lifestyle. Meals are viewed as social moments, encouraging people to slow down, enjoy their food, and connect with their community. This forms part of the Nordic concept of "hygge," a feeling of coziness and contentment. The sense of enjoyment associated with eating this way contributes to better mental and emotional well-being.

Busting Myths About the Nordic Diet

Despite its rising popularity, some misconceptions about the Nordic Diet persist. Let's address and debunk some of the most common myths:

Myth 1: "It's just a cold-climate Mediterranean Diet."

While there are some overlaps, the Nordic Diet's focus on local adaptability, foraged ingredients, and canola oil give it a unique identity. It is not simply a clone with different branding—it's tailored to the unique agricultural landscape and lifestyle of Nordic countries.

Myth 2: "It's too expensive to follow."

Many assume that eating organic or local always means spending more money. However, the Nordic Diet's preference for in-season produce and traditional food preparation methods makes it surprisingly affordable. Root vegetables, canned or smoked fish, and whole grains like barley are budget-friendly options that pack a nutritional punch.

Myth 3: "It's too restrictive."

On the contrary, the Nordic Diet provides immense variety. From plant-based soups and roasted vegetables to indulgent yogurt desserts topped with fresh berries, it allows for a broad spectrum of flavors and textures. The emphasis on balance, rather than cutting out complete food groups, ensures long-term adherence.

Myth 4: "It's not suitable for other climates or regions."

While its roots are in Scandinavia, the Nordic Diet's principles of sustainable and seasonal eating can be adapted anywhere in the world. People across different regions can easily replace specific Nordic staples like moss or lingonberries with local alternatives that fit their climate and agriculture.

The Nordic Diet is not just a trendy eating plan—it's a powerful framework for healthy and sustainable living. Its emphasis on local, seasonal foods; reliance on minimally processed ingredients; and culturally rich traditions make it a standout choice.

Whether for its proven health benefits or its eco-friendly approach, the Nordic Diet exemplifies how modern diets can be both mindful and enjoyable. By addressing misconceptions and showcasing its advantages, it's clear that Nordic eating is more than a fad—it's a lifestyle worth exploring.

Real-Life Testimonials

Clay Abney

Clay Abney's experience with the Nordic Diet in Norway highlights its health benefits and cultural richness. He found the diet, which emphasizes seafood, vegetables, and limiting processed foods, naturally packed with nutrients. His visit to Trondheim and the island of Hitra showcased sustainable practices, such as divers hand-picking scallops to protect ocean habitats. "Just like the Mediterranean diet, the Nordic diet is a very healthy way to eat," Clay shared. He also embraced the focus on seasonal, local foods, which ensures freshness and nutrition. Clay's experience revealed how this diet encourages not just healthy eating but also an active lifestyle.

Michelle King

Michelle King had a remarkable experience trying the Nordic diet for a week. She noticed a boost in both her mood and energy levels, saying, "Creating meals based around whole foods I enjoyed gave me more energy throughout the day." The emphasis on fresh, wholesome ingredients inspired her to cook at home more, which she truly enjoyed.

The meals, which included smoked salmon toast and lentil soup, were satisfying and delicious. By focusing on gut-friendly foods like fermented veggies and omega-3-rich fish, Michelle felt lighter and healthier. The Nordic diet left her feeling more connected to her food and overall happiness.

Tracy Partridge-Johnson

Tracy Partridge-Johnson found the Nordic diet to be a promising approach to eating healthier. She appreciated its balanced ratio of proteins, whole grains, and vegetables, saying, "The approach in this book sounds a little more balanced and less extreme." The diet's simplicity stood out, allowing her to include foods like oats, potatoes, berries, and nuts, which she enjoyed.

While noting a slight learning curve in balancing carbs and proteins, Tracy saw great potential in its scientifically-backed benefits for weight management and overall health. She viewed the diet as a practical, sustainable way to stay healthy without sacrificing variety.

7-Day Sample Meal Plan

Here's a 7-day sample meal plan inspired by the Nordic Diet, focusing on seasonal, local, and organic foods. Each day includes breakfast, lunch, dinner, and a snack, reflecting the balance and variety the diet offers.

Day 1

Breakfast: Rye Porridge with Fresh Berries

Lunch: Smoked Salmon on Dark Rye Bread

Dinner: Roasted Root Vegetable and Lentil Stew

Snack: Skyr with Lingonberry Jam

Day 2

Breakfast: Oat and Barley Muesli

Lunch: Nordic Herring Salad

Dinner: Mustard-Glazed Baked Salmon with Cabbage Slaw

Snack: Roasted Beet Chips and Hummus

Day 3

Breakfast: Buckwheat Pancakes with Berries

Lunch: Vegetable Soup with Quinoa

Dinner: Arctic Char with Dill-Potato Mash

Snack: Apple Slices with Almond Butter

Day 4

Breakfast: Nordic-Style Overnight Oats

Lunch: Rye Bread with Beetroot Spread and Avocado

Dinner: Braised Cabbage with Wild Game Meatballs

Snack: Rye Crispbread with Goat Cheese

Day 5

Breakfast: Barley Porridge with Cinnamon

Lunch: Nordic Fish Soup

Dinner: Dill-Marinated Chicken with Roasted Vegetables

Snack: Fresh Pear with Walnuts

Day 6

Breakfast: Skyr and Berries Bowl

Lunch: Nordic Bean Salad

Dinner: Baked Mackerel with Barley Pilaf

Snack: Pickled Cucumbers and Hard-Boiled Egg

Day 7

Breakfast: Smoked Trout on Crispbread

Lunch: Wild Mushroom and Spinach Barley Risotto

Dinner: Mustard-Crusted Cod with Root Veggie Mash

Snack: Roasted Nuts and Berries

This meal plan embraces the key principles of the Nordic Diet while offering diverse and flavorful options that are easy to prepare and delightful to eat.

Sample Recipes

We have included a few sample recipes below to give you an idea of the types of meals you can enjoy on this meal plan. Don't be afraid to get creative and add your own spin to these dishes!

Nordic Fish Soup

Ingredients:

- 1 pound white fish fillets, such as cod or haddock
- 2 tablespoons butter
- 1 leek, chopped
- 2 carrots, peeled and chopped
- 2 celery stalks, chopped
- 8 cups fish stock or vegetable broth
- 1 teaspoon dried dill
- Salt and pepper to taste

Instructions:

1. In a large pot over medium heat, melt the butter.
2. Add the leek, carrots, and celery and cook until softened, about 5 minutes.
3. Add the fish stock or broth and bring to a boil.
4. Reduce heat to low and let simmer for about 20 minutes.
5. Add the fish fillets and dill to the pot and let cook for an additional 10 minutes.
6. Season with salt and pepper, as desired.
7. Serve hot, garnished with fresh dill if desired.

Wild Mushroom and Spinach Barley Risotto

Ingredients:

- 1 cup barley
- 4 cups vegetable broth
- 2 tbsp olive oil
- 1 onion, chopped
- 2 cloves garlic, minced
- 1 lb mixed wild mushrooms, sliced
- 2 cups baby spinach leaves
- Salt and pepper, to taste

Instructions:

1. In a large pot, bring vegetable broth to a simmer.
2. In a separate pan, heat olive oil over medium heat and add onion and garlic. Cook until softened.
3. Add barley to the pan with the onions and garlic and toast for about 5 minutes.
4. Gradually add the hot broth to the barley mixture, stirring constantly until all liquid is absorbed and barley is tender.
5. In a separate pan, sauté the mushrooms until softened and add them to the barley mixture.
6. Stir in baby spinach leaves and season with salt and pepper to taste.
7. Serve hot and enjoy!

Baked Mackerel with Barley Pilaf

Ingredients:

- 4 mackerel fillets
- Salt and pepper, to taste
- 2 tbsp olive oil
- 1 onion, chopped
- 2 cloves garlic, minced
- 1 cup pearl barley
- 2 cups vegetable broth
- 1 lemon, sliced for garnish

Instructions:

1. Preheat oven to 375°F (190°C).
2. Season the mackerel fillets with salt and pepper on both sides.
3. In a large pan over medium heat, heat olive oil and add onions and garlic. Cook until softened.
4. Add in the pearl barley and stir until coated with oil.
5. Pour in the vegetable broth and bring to a boil. Once boiling, reduce heat and let simmer for 30 minutes.
6. In a separate pan, cook mackerel fillets until golden brown on both sides.
7. Serve the cooked barley pilaf as a bed for the baked mackerel fillets, and garnish with lemon slices.
8. Enjoy your delicious and healthy meal!

Oat and Barley Muesli

Ingredients:

- 1 cup rolled oats
- 1 cup barley flakes
- 2 tbsp honey or maple syrup
- 1/4 cup dried cranberries
- 1/4 cup chopped almonds
- 1 tsp ground cinnamon
- Milk or yogurt, for serving

Instructions:

1. In a large mixing bowl, combine rolled oats and barley flakes.
2. Add in honey or maple syrup and mix well to coat the grains.
3. Stir in dried cranberries, chopped almonds, and ground cinnamon.
4. Serve with milk or yogurt as desired.
5. Enjoy your nutritious oat and barley muesli for breakfast!

Barley Porridge

Ingredients:

- 2 cups cooked barley
- 1/2 cup milk
- 2 tsp. brown sugar
- 1/4 tsp. cinnamon
- 2 tbsp. walnuts, chopped and toasted
- fresh banana, sliced
- heavy cream

Instructions:

1. Put the barley, brown sugar, milk, and cinnamon in a saucepan over medium heat.
2. Cook the mixture for about 15 minutes, or until the barley has absorbed almost all the liquid.
3. Ladle the porridge into individual serving bowls.
4. Top each bowl with a banana and walnuts.
5. Drizzle heavy cream over the topping.
6. Serve and enjoy.

Thai-Style Chicken Pizza

Ingredients:

- 8 oz. pizza dough
- 1 cup roast chicken, shredded
- 3/4 cup red Thai curry sauce
- 5-1/2 cups carrots, shredded
- 1/2 cup red bell pepper, thin slices
- half of a small red onion, thinly sliced
- 1/4 cup Monterey jack cheese, shredded
- fresh cilantro

Instructions:

1. Preheat your oven to 525°F.
2. Put the pizza dough on a lightly floured surface. Roll it out until it becomes a very thin oval or rectangle measuring about 15" x 11."
3. Put the pizza dough on a baking sheet.
4. Put the curry sauce on the pizza dough and spread it evenly to cover the entire dough, including the edges.
5. Sprinkle the remaining ingredients, except the cilantro, on the dough.
6. Put the pizza in the oven and bake for 8 to 10 minutes until the dough turns crisp and golden.
7. Top the pizza with fresh cilantro just before serving.

Black Bean Burger

Ingredients:

- 16-oz. can black beans
- 1 pc. yellow onion, chopped
- 1/4 cup parsley, chopped
- 1 clove garlic, minced
- 1 tsp. ground cumin
- 1/2 tsp. kosher salt
- 1/2 tsp. black pepper
- 1 tbsp. canola oil
- 5 oz. peas and carrots
- 3/4 cup panko
- large egg
- 4 or 5 pcs. whole wheat rolls
- tomato slices, for garnish
- white onion slices, for garnish
- shredded lettuce, for garnish
- ketchup
- mustard

Instructions:

1. Rinse and drain the black beans.
2. Using a food processor, puree half of the black beans together with the parsley, onion, salt, pepper, and cumin until the mixture is smooth.

3. Turn the pureed burger mixture into a large bowl. Combine with the remaining half of the beans, carrots, peas, panko, and egg.
4. Form the patties. Make about 4 or 5 patties.
5. Heat the oil in a skillet.
6. Put the patties in the skillet and cook for about 3 to 4 minutes until they turn golden brown.
7. Flip the patties and continue cooking for another 3 to 4 minutes until cooked through.
8. Put one patty on each whole-wheat roll.
9. Garnish with tomato, onion, and lettuce. Add ketchup and mustard if desired.

Cocoa Oatmeal with Toasted Almonds and Coconut

Ingredients:

- 4 cups coconut milk
- 2 cups quick-cooking oats
- 1/4 cup unsweetened cocoa powder
- 1/4 tsp. salt
- flaked coconut, toasted
- chopped almonds, toasted
- optional: maple syrup

Instructions:

1. In a medium saucepan, bring the coconut milk to a boil.
2. Add the cocoa powder, salt, and oats. Stir.
3. Let the mixture boil again then bring down the heat.
4. Let the mixture simmer for a couple of minutes until it thickens.
5. Ladle the mixture into individual serving bowls.
6. Top each bowl with toasted almonds and flaked coconut.
7. Upon serving, add a drizzle of maple syrup if desired.

Baked Spanish Mackerel Filets

Ingredients:

- 6 pcs. Spanish mackerel filets
- 1/4 cup canola oil
- salt
- ground black pepper
- paprika
- 12 slices lemon

Instructions:

1. Arrange the oven rack so that it lies around 6 inches away from the source of heat.
2. Preheat the oven to 500°F.
3. Get a baking dish and lightly grease it.
4. Prepare each mackerel by rubbing both sides with canola oil.
5. Season the filets with salt, pepper, and paprika.
6. Top each filet with a couple of lemon slices.
7. Bake the filets for about 5 to 7 minutes, or just until the fish starts to flake.
8. Serve the fish right away.

Braised Cabbage

Ingredients:

- 1 tbsp. canola oil
- 1 tbsp. butter
- 1 small head red cabbage, sliced thinly
- salt
- 1/3 cup water,
- 1/4 cup red wine
- 2 tbsp. red wine vinegar
- 2 tbsp. honey
- caraway seeds

Instructions:

1. Heat the canola oil in a large skillet.
2. Add the butter and let it melt.
3. Add the cabbage. Cook for 1 or 2 minutes until the cabbage becomes soft.
4. Season the cabbage with salt.
5. Add the water, red wine vinegar, and wine. Stir to blend.
6. Add the honey and the caraway seeds.
7. Continue cooking for about 5 minutes more to allow the liquid to evaporate and the cabbage to become tender. Add more water if necessary.

Vegetable Omelet

Ingredients:

- 2 pcs. large eggs
- 1/4 cup bell pepper, chopped
- 1/4 cup mushrooms, chopped
- 2 tbsp. red onion, chopped
- 1/2 cup cherry tomatoes, chopped
- 1/2 cup fresh spinach, chopped
- salt
- pepper
- 2 tbsp. fresh parsley
- apple slices, for serving
- pear slices, for serving

Instructions:

1. Combine all the chopped vegetables and set aside.
2. Beat the eggs.
3. Add the vegetables to the beaten eggs.
4. Get a medium-sized skillet. Turn the heat to medium-high and pour the beaten eggs into the skillet.
5. Cook the mixture for 2 or 3 minutes or until the edges of the omelet are brown.

6. Flip the omelet over. Continue cooking for another 2 or 3 minutes.
7. Sprinkle salt and pepper to taste. Add parsley. Garnish with sliced onion.
8. Serve with apple or pear slices on the side.

Chicken in Bouillon

Ingredients:

- 6 pcs. chicken legs
- 2 tbsp. canola oil
- 2 shallot stalks, chopped finely
- 2 tsp. fennel seeds
- 1 cup apple juice
- 2-1/2 cups chicken stock
- 2 cups wheat grains or rye, spelled, or polished barley, rinsed well
- 2-1/2 cups green asparagus, each one cut into 4 pieces
- 2-1/2 cups spinach, chopped roughly
- salt
- pepper

For the gastrique:

- 4 cups balsamic vinegar
- 1 cup brown sugar

Instructions:

1. To prepare the gastrique, use a heavy-bottom saucepan to caramelize the sugar. Add the balsamic vinegar. Let the caramel dissolve.
2. When the mixture becomes syrupy in consistency, transfer it to a bottle. Keep the bottle in the refrigerator.
3. Sauté the chicken legs until they turn golden brown.

4. Put in the apple juice, fennel seeds, and shallots. Cook for around 2 minutes.
5. Put in the stock. Bring the mixture to a boil.
6. Bring down the heat and let the mixture simmer for 30 minutes.
7. Put them in another pan and let them simmer for about 12 minutes.
8. Add the wheat grains to the chicken.
9. Put in the asparagus.
10. Season the mixture with salt and pepper.
11. Add gastrique according to your taste. Let the mixture simmer for 8 to 10 minutes.
12. Add the spinach just before serving.

Grilled Halibut Niçoise with Mixed Vegetables

Ingredients:

- 4 pcs. large eggs
- 1-1/2 lb. halibut filets, skin on
- 1/4 cup plus 2 tbsp. canola oil
- salt
- pepper
- 2 lbs. mixed vegetables in season, like romano beans, scallions, new potatoes, halved small eggplants, and garlic flower buds
- 4 cups red leaf, butter, or romaine lettuce, torn
- 1 cup tomatoes, halved
- 1 bunch small breakfast radishes, trimmed and halved lengthwise
- 1 cup green olive tapenade

Instructions:

1. Boil water. Add the eggs and cook for about 7 minutes.
2. Put the eggs in ice water to cool.
3. Put the grill on medium-high heat.
4. Use 2 tablespoons of the oil to rub on the halibut.
5. Season the filets with salt and pepper according to taste.
6. Put the filets, skin side down, on the grill.
7. Grill for between 5 to 8 minutes or until the skin is charred and the filets are cooked through.

8. Turn the filets and continue cooking for a minute more.

9. Remove the filets from the grill and put them on a plate.

10. Take the charred skin out. Set the fish aside.

11. In a large bowl, toss the mixed vegetables in the remaining canola oil. Add salt and pepper to season.

12. Grill the vegetables. Turn occasionally. The vegetables will cook at different times.

13. Transfer the vegetables to a plate when they are done, tender and a bit charred.

14. Peel and halve the eggs.

15. Put the halibut filets, radishes, tomatoes, eggs, and grilled vegetables on a bed of lettuce leaves.

16. Drizzle green olive tapenade over the fish and vegetables.

17. Serve some of the tapenade on the side.

Sautéed Pineapple and Yogurt

Ingredients:

- 8-10 oz. fresh pineapple, cut into cubes
- 1 tbsp. honey
- 1/4 tsp. cinnamon
- 1/4 cup orange juice
- 3 cups yogurt, fat-free, plain
- 4 tbsp. pistachios, unsalted and chopped

Instructions:

1. Use medium-high heat to heat a large skillet. Cover the skillet with a light coating of cooking spray.
2. Put in the cubed pineapple, cinnamon, and honey. Stir. Let the mixture simmer for about a minute.
3. Add the orange juice. Cook for about 3 to 4 minutes so that the fruit absorbs the flavors and the sauce thickens a bit.
4. Serve the yogurt in individual serving bowls.
5. Top each bowl with the sautéed pineapple. Garnish with chopped pistachios.

Steamed Cauliflower and Curried Shrimp

Ingredients:

- 1 whole cauliflower, separated into florets
- 2 tbsp. canola oil
- 2 cloves garlic, minced
- 1 cup sweet peppers, chopped finely
- 1 lb. bay shrimps, pre-cooked
- 1 tsp. curry powder
- 1 tsp. butter
- 3 tbsp. flour
- 1/2 cup fish or vegetable broth
- 2/3 cup milk, low-fat
- 1 tbsp. fresh dill, finely chopped
- 1/4 cup pine nuts, toasted

Instructions:

1. Steam the cauliflower until tender. Set aside.
2. Use a frying pan to sauté the garlic. Add the peppers. Continue cooking until the peppers start to soften.
3. Add the curry powder and the shrimp. Remove pan from heat and set aside.
4. Prepare the roux. Melt the butter. Add the flour and whisk. Heat until the roux becomes light golden brown.
5. Add the milk and broth to the roux gradually. Whisk to incorporate. Stir constantly until the sauce starts to bubble.

6. Add the curried shrimp. Bring the heat down and cook for another 5 minutes.
7. Toss the cauliflower in the shrimp sauce.
8. Transfer to a serving platter. Garnish with dill and pine nuts.

Seared Salmon

Ingredients:

- 1-1/2 tbsp. canola oil
- 4 pcs. salmon filets, each filet about 1-inch thick
- 1 tsp. kosher salt
- 1 tsp. ground black pepper, 1 teaspoon
- 2/3 cups shallots, thinly sliced, 2/3 cup
- 3 cups cherry tomatoes, 3 cups
- 2 tbsp. balsamic vinegar
- 1/2 cup basil leaves, torn

Instructions:

1. Preheat the oven to 500°F.
2. Use foil when lining a rimmed baking sheet, then set aside.
3. Put a tablespoon of canola oil in a large heavy-bottomed pan placed over high heat.
4. Sprinkle evenly half of the pepper and salt over the fish filets.
5. Cook the filets in the pan for 4 minutes until the sides are golden brown.
6. Transfer the filets, with seared sides up, onto the prepared baking sheet.
7. Put it in the oven and cook the filet for about 4 minutes or until you get the degree of doneness that you prefer.

8. Return the skillet to the stove, and add the remaining canola oil.

9. Add the shallots and sauté for a couple of minutes. Season with the remaining salt and pepper.

10. Add the cherry tomatoes and 1/3 cup basil. Cook until the tomatoes are soft, for about 2 minutes.

11. Add the balsamic vinegar. Stir and cook for about a minute.

12. Transfer the filets to a serving dish and top with the balsamic vinegar-tomato mixture. Garnish with the remaining basil.

13. Serve and enjoy while hot.

Barley Oat Pancakes

Ingredients:

- 1 cup barley flour
- 1 cup oat flour
- 1 tbsp. baking powder, sodium-free
- 1 tsp. salt
- 1-1/2 cup nonfat milk
- 2 pcs. large eggs
- 2 tbsp. canola oil
- 2 tbsp. honey
- 2 tsp. vanilla extract
- honey or maple syrup, for serving
- your choice of fresh fruit

Instructions:

1. In a large mixing bowl, whisk together the oat flour, barley flour, salt, and baking powder.
2. In a separate mixing bowl, whisk together the eggs, oil, non-fat milk, vanilla extract, and honey.
3. Transfer the wet ingredients to the large mixing bowl. Whisk them together to combine. Do not overmix the batter.
4. Place a large non-stick pan over low-medium heat.
5. Put about 3 tablespoons of batter into the pan. Wait for bubbles to appear on the top side of the pancake and the bottom to turn golden brown.

6. Flip the pancake to cook the other side.

7. Repeat until all the batter is cooked.

8. Top each pancake with your choice of fresh fruit.

9. Drizzle honey or maple syrup over the fruit.

10. Serve the pancakes immediately.

Roast Broccoli and Salmon

Ingredients:

- 1 bunch broccoli, cut into florets
- 4 tbsp. canola oil, divided
- salt
- pepper
- 4 pcs. salmon filets, skins removed
- 1 pc. jalapeño or red Fresno chile, seeds removed, sliced into thin rings
- 2 tbsp. rice vinegar, unseasoned
- 2 tbsp. capers, drained

Instructions:

1. Preheat the oven to 400° F.
2. On a large, rimmed baking sheet, put the broccoli florets and toss in 2 tablespoons of the canola oil. Season with salt and pepper.
3. Roast the florets in the oven for 12 or 15 minutes. Toss occasionally.
4. Remove from the oven when the florets are crisp-tender and browned.
5. Gently rub the filets with 1 tablespoon of the canola oil. Season the salmon with salt and pepper.
6. Put the salmon in the middle of the baking sheet.

7. Move the florets to the sides of the baking sheet. Roast the filet for 10 to 15 minutes or until the filets turn opaque throughout.

8. In a small bowl, combine the vinegar, chile rings, and a pinch of salt.

9. Let the mixture sit for about 10 minutes so that the chile rings become somewhat softened,

10. Add the capers and the remaining tablespoon of canola oil. Add salt and pepper to taste.

11. Drizzle chile vinaigrette over the roasted broccoli and salmon just before serving.

Carrot Soup

Ingredients:

- 8 pcs. carrots, chopped roughly
- half an onion, chopped roughly
- 1 apple, chopped
- 1/4 tsp. ground cumin
- 1/2 cup apple cider
- 1/2 cup whole milk or light cream
- salt
- pepper

Instructions:

1. Put the carrots and onions in a saucepan. Cover with enough water.
2. Cook until soft.
3. Add the apple slices. Continue cooking until the apple becomes soft and tender.
4. Transfer the mixture to a food processor or blender. Puree.
5. Return the pureed mixture to the saucepan.
6. Add the milk, apple cider, and cumin. Add salt and pepper to taste.
7. Heat the soup until hot. Do not allow it to boil.
8. Add more cider for a thinner soup.
9. Serve and enjoy while hot.

Braised Red Cabbage

Ingredients:

- 1/8 tsp. caraway seeds
- 2 tbsp. white sugar
- 2 tbsp. red wine vinegar
- 2 tbsp. red wine
- 1/4 cup of red wine
- 1/3 cup of water
- 1 red cabbage, cored and thinly sliced into strips
- 2 tbsp. butter

Instructions:

1. Preheat a skillet over low-medium heat.
2. Melt 2 tbsp. butter, stirring it in random circular motions to evenly spread it on the pan.
3. Sauté cabbage slices for a minute. Season with a pinch of salt, and pour the red wine, water, and vinegar. Stir to combine with a wooden spatula.
4. Stir in the caraway seeds and sugar. Keep mixing until the veggies are tender and the sauce has evaporated. It may take about 5 minutes to cook the cabbage slices.
5. Transfer the contents of the pan onto a serving dish.
6. Serve and enjoy while hot.

Nordic Maple Syrup

Ingredients:

- salt
- 1/4 tsp. nutmeg
- 1 cinnamon stick
- 2 tbsp. maple syrup
- 3 tbsp. water
- 2-1/2 lb. apples, cored, deseeded, and quartered

Instructions:

1. In a pressure cooker, combine the nutmeg, cinnamon stick, maple syrup, water, and apple slices.
2. Cook on high heat for eight minutes. Let the pressure build for about 12 minutes.
3. When done, use the natural method to release pressure.
4. After half an hour, unlock the lid and remove it.
5. Throw out the cinnamon stick and drizzle a pinch of salt.
6. To attain your desired consistency, blend the mixture with an immersion blender.

Conclusion

Thank you for taking the time to explore this guide to the Nordic Diet. By reaching this point, you've made a meaningful commitment to learning about a lifestyle that celebrates simplicity, sustainability, and your well-being. Whether you're already preparing to stock your pantry with rye bread and root vegetables or simply considering small changes, you're on the path to creating a healthier, more mindful way of living.

The Nordic Diet isn't just another fleeting food trend—it's a philosophy rooted in balance, tradition, and thoughtful choices. This diet invites you to slow down, take notice of what you put on your plate, and connect to the natural rhythms of the seasons. Unlike rigid meal plans or complicated rules, the Nordic Diet offers flexibility. Its core principle is simple yet profound: prioritize fresh, local, and nutrient-rich ingredients. This isn't about deprivation; it's about abundance and making room for wholesome, delicious foods that both nourish you and honor the environment.

One of the most remarkable aspects of the Nordic lifestyle is how sustainable it is. By eating seasonally and sourcing your food locally when possible, you reduce your environmental footprint and support the farmers in your community. Imagine the impact you could make by not only investing in your health but also contributing to a more sustainable planet. Every choice you make around food ripples out, creating change far beyond your dining table.

The Nordic Diet also makes exploring health and wellness feel attainable. It doesn't call for calorie counting, rigid restrictions, or exclusive superfoods. Instead, you're encouraged to enjoy everyday ingredients that are easy to find—berries bursting with flavor, hearty root vegetables, omega-3-rich fish, and aromatic herbs and spices. These are not only delicious but also packed with essential nutrients that fuel your body and keep you energized.

Perhaps the best part of this lifestyle is its focus on mindfulness and connection. The Nordic Diet encourages you to prepare meals at home, sit down at the table, and savor each bite. It celebrates quality time shared with loved ones over nourishing dishes, creating not just meals but meaningful moments. It reminds you that eating well is about more than health—it's about happiness, too.

If the idea of shifting your habits and adopting a new approach to eating feels overwhelming, take a deep breath and remember that change happens step by step. Start small. Replace a refined grain with a whole grain. Cook with seasonal vegetables this week. Swap one processed snack for a homemade treat. Every small shift counts, and before you know it, these changes will feel like second nature.

The Nordic Diet isn't a quick fix or a temporary solution; it's a lifestyle. It's about choosing health, kindness to the planet, and intention in how you nourish yourself. Most importantly, it's something you can sustain for the long haul—because it's delicious, it feels good, and it's simple enough to stick with.

Now it's your turn. Take what you've learned here and bring it to life in your kitchen, your community, and your mindset. Explore the flavors, experiment with the recipes, and make them your own. The Nordic Diet is a gift for your well-being—but it's also a gift you share with the world by practicing sustainability and mindfulness. Start today, and enjoy the transformation ahead.

FAQs

What is the Nordic Diet, and how does it differ from other eating plans?

The Nordic Diet is inspired by the traditional foods of Nordic countries like Denmark, Sweden, Norway, Finland, and Iceland. It emphasizes local, seasonal, and sustainable foods, such as whole grains, root vegetables, berries, fatty fish, and canola oil. Unlike many diets, it focuses on simplicity, balance, and environmental consciousness. While similar to the Mediterranean Diet, it prioritizes Nordic-specific ingredients (like rye, barley, and herring) and uses canola oil instead of olive oil as a key source of healthy fats.

What are the health benefits of following the Nordic Diet?

The Nordic Diet is linked to numerous health benefits, such as improved heart health, better digestion, and reduced inflammation. It also aids in weight management due to its focus on nutrient-dense, high-fiber foods that promote satiety. Additionally, studies have shown it can lower blood pressure, cholesterol levels, and the risk of chronic diseases like type-2 diabetes. The inclusion of omega-3-rich fish and antioxidant-loaded berries further enhances overall health.

How can I start adopting the Nordic Diet?

To begin, focus on incorporating more whole, seasonal, and locally sourced ingredients into your meals. Start with simple swaps, like replacing refined grains with whole grains like rye or oats, using canola oil instead of butter, and including more root vegetables and fatty fish. Visit farmer's markets for fresh, seasonal produce and consider joining a CSA program. Gradually reduce processed foods and sugary snacks, and aim to cook meals at home to control ingredients and savor the process.

Do I need to give up meat to follow the Nordic Diet?

No, the Nordic Diet is not vegetarian or vegan. While it emphasizes plant-based meals, moderate amounts of meat, particularly wild game and lean options like chicken, are included. The diet also champions fish and seafood as primary protein sources due to their omega-3 content. Meat is typically treated as a complementary ingredient rather than the focal point of meals, promoting balance and sustainability.

Is the Nordic Diet expensive to follow?

Not necessarily. While organic or local ingredients might seem pricier upfront, seasonal produce, whole grains, and canned or smoked fish (like mackerel or sardines) are often affordable.

Additionally, the diet encourages reducing food waste and preparing meals at home, which can save money in the long run. Foraging for local ingredients, if possible, and buying in bulk (e.g., grains and legumes) can further minimize costs.

What are the most common misconceptions about the Nordic Diet?

One common misconception is that the Nordic Diet is restrictive, but it's actually quite flexible and includes a variety of ingredients. Another myth is that it's designed solely for cold climates—its core principles of seasonal and local eating can be adapted anywhere in the world. Additionally, some assume it's expensive, but its focus on simplicity, seasonal produce, and whole grains makes it accessible on a budget.

How can I incorporate the Nordic Diet into my daily routine?

Start small by incorporating one Nordic-inspired meal each day. For example, have oatmeal with berries for breakfast, a leafy green salad with rye crispbread for lunch, or roasted root veggies and baked salmon for dinner. Simplify your cooking techniques by roasting, boiling, or baking ingredients to highlight their natural flavors. Focus on eating mindfully—share meals with loved ones and avoid distractions like TV while eating. Gradually, these habits will help you fully integrate the Nordic Diet into your lifestyle.

References and Helpful Links

Harvard Health. (2015, November 19). The Nordic diet: Healthy eating with an eco-friendly bent. https://www.health.harvard.edu/blog/the-nordic-diet-healthy-fare-with-an-eco-friendly-bent-201511198673

Garone, S. (2021, January 12). Eating Nordic Won't Turn You into a Viking, but It Might Transform How You Feel. Greatist. https://greatist.com/eat/nordic-diet

McKay, A. (2022, March 23). The Nordic Diet: How to eat like a Scandinavian. Life in Norway. https://www.lifeinnorway.net/nordic-diet/

BSc, K. G. (2023b, November 10). Mediterranean Diet 101: A Meal Plan and Beginner's guide. Healthline. https://www.healthline.com/nutrition/mediterranean-diet-meal-plan

Clinic, C. (2024a, August 12). Nordic diet: What is it and what can you eat? Cleveland Clinic. https://health.clevelandclinic.org/nordic-diet

Ms, J. L. (2019, February 27). The Nordic Diet: An Evidence-Based Review. Healthline. https://www.healthline.com/nutrition/the-nordic-diet-review#:~:text=The%20bottom%20line,evidence%20is%20weak%20and%20inconsistent.

What's the Nordic diet? (n.d.). WebMD. https://www.webmd.com/diet/ss/slideshow-nordic-diet#:~:text=This%20style%20of%20eating%20is,seas%2C%20lakes%2C%20and%20the%20wild

9 781795 781534